Exercises for Eating Mindfully Volume Five

Mindfulness Practices for Persons with Parkinson's Disease

9/3/2014
Parkinsons Recovery
Robert Rodgers PhD

Contents

© Parkinsons Recovery

The Parkinsons Recovery Mindfulness Series

Realistically speaking, how can the intense level of stress that aggravates the symptoms of Parkinson's disease be calmed? Better yet, how can they be quieted? My research over the past decade reveals that using your mind to drop the stress level down a notch or two always backfires. When you tell yourself:

- *Settle down!*
- *Take it easy!*
- *Stop being so stressed out!*

The stress level ratchets up, not down. Attempts to force the stress and anxiety levels to adjust downward induce an internally generated stress. They pile more stress on top of an excess of stress that already exists. There are certainly a sufficient number of external generators of stress in every one's life. Why infuse more stress that you create yourself, even with the best of intentions?

If the mind is not a useful technique to reduce stress, what is? The most eloquent answer I have for you is to become more mindful of what is experienced in the present moment. Becoming more mindful shifts you into the experience of the "now" which in itself is less stressful (unless you have been kidnapped by terrorists!).

It is stressful to anticipate events you imagine will occur in the future. The events we imagine rarely happen. Does this ring true for you? We all create unnecessary stress in our lives by how and where we focus our thoughts and attention.

It is stressful to agonize over the past. When we think about the past, we are much more likely to think about unpleasant experiences that induce stress. The past event itself was traumatic enough. Yet, we insist on reliving the trauma over and over again through our memories. It seems some of us just can't get enough stress in our lives.

The problem with upping the ante on stress levels is that – as you well know – symptoms of Parkinson's disease become worse. When you are not as stressed, your symptoms are far less problematic.

I have reached one solid conclusion from my ten years of research on Parkinson's disease. Symptoms will drive you crazy when you are stressed and are far less problematic when stress is under control.

Now, if you can't use your mind to become more mindful (which creates added stress in itself) how in the world can you quiet down a frantic lifestyle? I have concluded that the simplest and most effective solution to reducing stress levels is to become more mindful.

The transformation is possible step by step through these simple exercises you can do anywhere, anytime of the day. The Parkinsons Recovery mindfulness exercises are designed to focus your attention on the present moment as attention on either the past or the future is diverted. A renewed focus on the present moment reduces stress levels. Mindfulness is a lifestyle that will reduce stresses in your life if you set the intention to take a mindfulness practice seriously.

I recommend that you practice each of the exercises for a week or longer. Incorporate each practice into your regular routines and habits. Attempts to do all of the exercises simultaneously will likely induce more stress which – obviously – is contrary to the intent of a successful mindfulness program.

Give each exercise a little time and space. Invite the stresses in your life to dissipate. Allow the experience of each practice to engulf you. In so doing, watch the stresses in your life dip down to new lows along with a concurrent relief of any and all symptoms that you have currently been experiencing.

This volume is one out of nine I have developed to support the recovery of persons who currently experience neurological symptoms. A full listing of the Parkinsons Recovery Mindfulness themes follows:

Exercises for Eating Mindfully
Mindfulness Practices for Persons with Parkinson's Disease
Volume Five

Volume 1: Exercises for Seeing Mindfully

Volume 2: Exercises for Hearing Mindfully

Volume 3: Exercises for Noticing Mindfully

Volume 4: Exercises for Doing Mindfully

Volume 5: Exercises for Eating Mindfully

Volume 6: Exercises for Thinking Mindfully

Volume 7: Exercises for Feeling Mindfully

Volume 8: Exercises for Being Mindfully

Volume 9: Exercises for Intending Mindfully

Robert Rodgers, PhD

Parkinsons Recovery

www.parkinsonsrecovery.me

Olympia, Washington

Eating Mindfully

The mindfulness challenge this week will be admittedly be a horrendous undertaking for most of you if indeed you decide you would like to run with it. The challenge is simply this; when you eat or when you drink anything, just eat and just drink. Do nothing else at the same time.

What do you typically do when you actually eat something? Are you walking or driving or watching TV? Perhaps you are watching a movie or reading or working on the computer or texting someone? Many people like to eat when they listen to music or play video games. Do you eat when you exercise? What do you do typically when you eat? What do you do in addition to eating besides the simple act of placing food into your body?

For this week the challenge and the invitation is to remove all of those extra activities that you add to the activity of eating which involves consuming food and liquids. It goes without saying that many of us like to eat in the company of another person. We love to have conversations with those we love. Please do not eliminate that activity. But when you do talk with loved ones, stop eating. In other words, disentangle the two activities.

When you eat, focus your full attention on the food itself –

- *on the chewing*
- *on the taste*
- *on the sensations in your mouth*
- *on the feeling in your stomach*

Treasure each and every bite as if it were your last. Add no other activity as you eat. This may well add considerable time to how long it takes to finish a meal. If you have to eat and run, you will have to set aside this challenge temporarily.

Try it and see how this alters the entire experience of ingesting nutrition into that most precious, sacred body of yours.

Notice when your body likes the food you eat.

Notice when it does not like the food you eat.

When we notice, we become aware in the moment of precisely what our body needs to heal. If a cow can eat mindfully, so can we!

I have my fingers crossed that this challenge will not become too horrendous for you. But be warned, it will be difficult. You will likely be surprised at how often you do much more than simply eat. My favorite "add on" activity to eating is thinking. It is so easy to divert our attention from a place away from the most important activity of the day.

Deeper Meaning Behind Eating Mindfully

Many people view eating as a time-wasting activity. The idea is to eat food quickly so you can get on with the business of living your life. Eating takes time away from what you really want to accomplish during the day. Eating takes time away from earning money, from improving the quality of relationships with family and friends, from earning prizes and accolades and from manifesting our passions. In other words, eating is viewed as a time-wasting activity that is required because we simply happen to have a body that requires nutrition each and every day. We cannot keep going if we do not feed ourselves. It is all a very practical matter you see.

Does this describe in whole or part your approach to eating? Think about eating from an entirely fresh perspective. What if the most important and critical action you can take each and every day is to be totally and completely mindful for a mere 30 minutes? This one action will ensure your body will be brought back into a place of centeredness and balance, a place where neurological symptoms have great difficulty creeping in.

When many people eat, they actually swallow their -

Sorrow or

Guilt or

Anger or

Fear or

Anxiety or

All of the above

Some people swallow their past as they reflect on past experiences that were unpleasant. Other people anticipate and plan out the future when they eat. Still others like to mix and match. All three of these eating rituals allow us to "space out" when eating. The magic of the present moment is lost. The taste and succulence of each and every bite is missed.

Consider recovery from any neurological condition seriously (and particularly from a condition associated with the diagnosis of Parkinson's disease). What more critical action can be taken than to focus your full attention on what you are putting into our body and to be mindful of how you ingest each bite of food?

10

When we take medicines or supplements we are also eating! Do you like to get the business of swallowing medications over and done with? Is it an unpleasant duty to be tolerated? Most people just pop pills and that is the end of it.

I have a mindful ritual to suggest when you take medications or supplements. The ritual takes only 15 seconds. It is analogous to a blessing before you begin eating a meal. The practice has a profound impact on the effectiveness of whatever supplements or medications you might be currently taking. Try it out and you will see what I mean for yourself.

Place the supplement or medication into your hand. Say silently to yourself or out loud:

1. *"May this supplement (or medication) do for my body precisely what my body needs - no more and no less."*

2. *Pause.*

3. *Take a short breath.*

4. *Ingest the supplement or medication.*

In other words you ask that the medication or supplement do for your body precisely what it is that your body needs now, no more – that is, no side-effects – and no less – meaning that is it has precisely the effect that you intend for it to have. This practice insures that you treat your body's response to taking the supplement or medication with respect.

- *Be mindful with each and every bite you ingest if it is food.*
- *Be mindful when you take medicines and supplements.*
- *Be mindful when you drink liquids.*

Notice when you ingest anything and, at the very same time, do something else like talk on the phone or drive or walk. Catch yourself when you tag an extra activity along with eating.

When you realize you are doubling up and doing more than just eating - stop. Eliminate the other activity. Direct your full attention to eating. Be mindful of every aspect of the food you eat – its color, smell, taste, texture and feel. Be mindful of the liquids you drink – their color, viscosity and taste.

Notice how it feels to enter into that most precious, sacred vessel of yours – your human body. The body is precious. It is a miracle in the making. Treat it as such. May you have a magnificent week as you eat each bite of food mindfully.

Food Indulgences

The challenge that I extend to you this week is to become mindful of the signals that your body sends to you when you eat food that is good and nutritious for your body and when you eat food that is not nutritious and is not good for your body.

In order to be able to take the challenge this week and run with it, you will need to take a little extra action. I fully understand if some of you refuse to take on the mantle of the challenge this week, but let me explain it anyway by way of emphasizing the signals that your body sends to you when you are giving it the nutrition that it needs and when you are not.

What food do you eat that you know is bad for your body, that is unhealthy for your system? The foods that I know I love to eat but are bad for my health and wellness turn out to be chocolate (or vanilla milkshakes) and macaroni and cheese. Now, I make no bones about it; I love, absolutely love, to eat each of those foods. There is no doubt about the temporary pleasure I derive when I eat them. There is some trigger of pleasure that sets in that must come from a place long ago and far away.

Of course, once I finish eating those foods, it is also the case that I feel absolutely horrible. I get sleepy.

Sometimes I have to take a nap. I become depressed. I say to myself,

> *"Oh well, it was worth it, I haven't had macaroni and cheese and a chocolate milkshake for a long time and I loved eating it all."*

Of course when I really look at the decision that I made the pleasure winds up lasting a mere 10 or 15 minutes. The aftermath winds up lasting as long as one or two days. And yet, most of us continue to eat food that dampens our life force and deflates our overall health and wellness.

The challenge I offer to you this week is the following. I know that the foods that you probably truly love and know are not bad for you probably not macaroni and cheese and chocolate milkshakes, but I do know that you are well aware of foods that you absolutely love to eat, but try not to eat too frequently because you know they are not good for your body.

This week I give you permission to indulge in a food that you know is bad for your body. Choose at least one food that you know is not good for you and eat it! The additional challenge however is to make very careful notes about how you feel after you eat food that is yummy to your soul and yet bad for your body. In other words, eat the food mindfully. Taste it. Treasure it.

Maybe - just maybe - it is not giving the pleasure that you thought it would. Most importantly, monitor how your body feels after you eat. Monitor how you feel several hours after you eat, if not for the rest of the day.

Do this (if you wish to take on the challenge) just once. Obviously it is not a smart idea to eat food that you know is not good for you so I will fully understand if you decide to pass on this particular challenge.

Let a little time pass. The companion challenge that I extend to you is to eat nutritious food that you know is exactly what your body needs. Consider eating fresh, live food that contains vibrant colors. Sometimes nutritious foods come in the form of salads or perhaps smoothies; you know what food is good for your body. Select nutritious food to eat and follow the same process as you followed when you ate food that was bad for your body.

Eat it mindfully, taking notice of what it means to eat each and every bite. Then, track how your body feels moment to moment, 30 minutes, an hour, two hours afterward and for the rest of the day. Be mindful of the signals that your body sends to you.

You already know the foods that are bad for you and the foods that are good for you. That is what determined the selection of what you wanted to eat under each instance. The power of this exercise is to become much more aware of the consequences when you eat food that is not in your best and highest good. I suspect that you will be amazed and excited about how wonderful you feel and how much energy you have when you eat food that is in fact good for your body. You may also marvel at the difference between the two.

Of course it may be the case that when you are eating fresh food, it is not exactly your cup of tea as they say. It may taste more like medicine than yummy for your tummy goodies. It may not exactly be food that you would typically choose to eat during the day. It is not the steak and potatoes that many people love to eat for a meal. The reality is that fresh food, the food that has colors, the food that is live, is the food that your body needs in order to return to full health and wellness.

To summarize, you have an official invitation to indulge – some people might call this "sinning" – and you also have an invitation to have an experience of eating good food that will nourish your body. Contrast the two experiences. Become more mindful of the consequences of each and every bite that you take of the food that you choose to eat.

May you have an exciting and intriguing time as you challenge yourself this week with becoming more mindful of eating good and bad foods. Neurons are very sensitive tissues. They need a lot support to become healthy.

Deeper Meaning Behind Food Indulgences

There's no question about it. Our bodies need live, nutritious organic food to maintain health and wellness. Many people tell me,

> "I don't have the resources to purchase organic food. I can't buy all of that live food that you say is so good for me. My budget simply won't allow it."

That is a choice, a choice that many people make. It is also a choice to incur the costs of hospital visits and the consequences of illness as we age. You can choose to incur the costs up front when you are younger and maintain health and wellness throughout your entire life, or you can accept the consequences of medicines and hospitalizations as you get older.

I will say it again. It is a choice. No additional studies are required or needed to show people who eat healthy, nutritious food each and every day will be far, far healthier, more vibrant and less depressed than individuals who eat food that they may love, but is not the food that their body needs to maintain health and wellness.

I am certainly not saying anything you do not already know. You know that eating healthy food will make a

17

difference. But, let me offer to you another choice that many people, including myself make. This choice is to say,

> *"Hmm, I believe that I'm not getting enough calcium and pantothenic acid."*

Don't ask me to say what those reasons are. Sometimes I just get hunches. Sometimes a healthcare provider tells me,

> *"Huh, you're looking a little pink these days. What you really need is more vitamin C or pantothenic acid or calcium, or ..."*

And, I say to myself,

> *"Oh, my heavens, I think you're right. Pink means ..."*

I rush to the supplement store and purchase these specific supplements. I begin to take them. After a while I say to myself,

> *"Huh, I believe the pink is fading! Look at me, look at me. I'm so happy I made such a good decision."*

Now, these particular choices can also be quite wise and instrumental in helping us to return to health. I'm certainly

18

not arguing against supplements. Let me make, however, another argument.

Supplements are simply food. Food is a way that we can obtain all the nutrition that we actually need. If we eat nutritious food each and every day – I don't mean every week, I mean each and every day – you, nor I, nor anyone, would actually need to take any supplements whatsoever. No follow up is required. No consultations with healthcare providers are necessary. No one needs to look at us and say,

> *"Hmm, you're looking a little pink today. Everything okay?"*

The reality is that if we set into motion a habit of eating fresh, live, organic food each and every day, we have an excellent chance of not only maintaining health and wellness, but of reversing disease states.   Am I saying that you will be able to reverse the symptoms of Parkinson's by eating healthy food? Maybe. Maybe not. But, some people are accomplishing just that.

Some doctors argue it will still be necessary to take supplements because the overall quality of food that is available to us today (as compared to 100 years ago) has been seriously depleted due to pesticides and the overall deterioration of the soils.

I do know however that it will make a huge and significant impact on how you feel each and every day if you eat organic food that is fresh. I also know that more and more people are coming out with announcements that they were able to heal seriously debilitating conditions by simply changing their diets. These are people that went to all the best medical doctors and received all the best and cutting-edge treatments and found that none of that really seemed to help. What really helped was to change their habit of what they put inside their body.

As an end note to this discussion, I just want to plant a seed of an idea that you may find to be useful. I personally find it sometimes difficult to eat a lot of greens, a lot of salads. It has never been something that I find is enjoyable. What I have discovered is a new approach.

I go to my local co-op. I purchase lots of fresh vegetables that have many, many different colors. I put them in my bag. The purchase cost at our co-op is very, very modest and reasonable; far less than what I would have to pay at a regular grocery store.

I come home and on a regular basis we juice these vegetables, usually combining them together with some fruits that make the juice yummy and tasteful. We put lots of things into this juice every day. It is live food. I can simply drink this yummy energy drink that we make ourselves every day. I can then be sure that every day I am getting the live food that I actually need.

One of the challenges of juicing that I have had previously is to wash all the parts of the juicer. It tended to take 20 or 30 minutes. Since I had books to write I was not taking the time to wash my juicer, so I stopped doing juicing for a year or two.

We're back to doing it and have purchased something called a Vitamix which is a juicer that is easy to clean. Yes, it does cost a bit of money, but the truth of the matter is, my choice is to pay the money up front now so that I can maintain my health as I age or pay the money later when hospital visits would be required.

As you continue to consider the difference between eating food that is yummy to your tummy but not good for your body, versus food that is required for your body to maintain health and wellness realize that with each bite we have a choice about what we put in our body. Every bite is a choice as to how we want to live and feel; the next hour, the next day, the next month and the next year and for the rest of our lives. Each mouth full is a choice.

I invite you to consider making new choices about what you eat if, in your own estimation, some of what you are eating is not in your best and highest good.

Be Mindful of Your Stomach

The mindfulness challenge this week is to pay particular and mindful attention to a most important organ of your body—your stomach.

1. **Pay attention to how your stomach feels before you eat anything.**
2. **Pay attention while you are eating something.**
3. **Pay attention after you have finished eating.**

How does your stomach feel across those three points in time? Before you begin eating, how does your stomach really feel? Are you really hungry before you eat?

As you eat, pay close attention to how your stomach actually feels. What are the sensations?

- *Are you eating until you are completely bloated and full?*
- *Are you eating only a little and not satisfying that hunger need which resides within your stomach?*
- *How does your stomach actually feel as you eat?*

Afterward - just few minutes afterward - how does your stomach feel? What are the sensations that you connect in with after you finish eating?

Be mindful. Focus on that most important digestive organ. See what valuable information comes through. Most of us are habitually ignorant of how our stomach sends signals that we need to eat or do not need to eat.

What information are you missing? You'll get it when you become mindful of precisely how your stomach is feeling in the moment.

Have a magnificent week as you pay close attention to the process of eating and ingesting food which resides happily inside your body.

Deeper Implications Behind Becoming Mindful of Your Stomach

What have you learned about yourself after becoming mindful of the sensations in your stomach as you ate a meal? Some people discover that their habit has been to eat upon first arising in the morning because that is what they were taught to do when they were kids. However, it is possible that the better time for you and your body to ingest food is much later on in the morning, like 11 or even 12.

Or, perhaps you always wait until 10:00 am to eat something. It is possible that the best strategy for you is to eat something immediately after popping up out of bed.

You will know the best time to eat first thing in the morning by listening carefully and connecting in with the sensations that your stomach sends out to you. Become mindful of your eating habits. It is possible that your long established habits of eating are not in tune with the needs of your body. Some people need to graze throughout the day. The idea of having two or three full meals is simply not well-suited to the needs of their body. Everybody is different.

Research clearly shows that the less that we eat, the longer we live and the happier our body actually is. There is a saying that if we stop eating when we are four-fifths full, we will maintain a state of continual balance and wellness. If we, as a habit, eat until we are full; that last fourth or fifth of food will guarantee that we are feeding our doctors and our healthcare professionals. We don't need to eat until we are totally full. Our stomach – and the sensations therein – tell us when to stop eating. We just have to pay attention and become mindful!

Being mindful of the sensations in the stomach, then, yields incredible insights about what our bodies need from us. Believe it or not, there are mindfulness workshops that involve the challenge of eating one single raisin. The task is to take time to connect in with the texture, the flavor, the aroma, the temperature and the color of the raisin. Many people who attend those workshops report a great surprise with the realization that they are full after eating one single raisin. Why is that the case? It's because they have engaged the full experience of pleasure in eating rather than simply crunching down food mouthful after mouthful without being mindful of the full experience of the:

- *colors*
- *smells*
- *temperature*
- *flavors*
- *textures*

Of the food we choose to eat and place inside our body.

A second most important reason to be mindful of the sensations in our stomach is that many people confuse anxiety and loneliness with being physically hungry. If we really connect with our stomach and the sensations that our stomach sends to us, we can disengage the feelings of anxiety from the sensations of hunger. Clearly, it is not going to help the anxiety if we try to override that with eating when the body does not need to be fed. Similarly, it is not going to help loneliness to over eat. The loneliness will still be present.

A resolution for both challenges is to be mindful of each and every bite that we take of the food that we choose to eat. To be mindful of the true essence of what it is that we put into our body, to acknowledge the difference between food that is live and food that is dead; to acknowledge and honor the difference between food that nourishes our body and food that damages our body. Once that food reaches our stomach, we know the difference because the sensations of our stomach will tell us what our body needs to nourish us back to health.

Many blessings and may you have a marvelous time as you continue to be mindful of the sensations in your stomach before you eat, during the course of eating and after you eat, always asking the questions -

1. **What's there?**
2. **Am I too full?**

3. **Am I not full enough?**

4. **Did I eat when I was hungry?**

Or, did I eat for other reasons, because -

- *I was anxious*
- *I was afraid*
- *I was lonely*

Disengaging the motivation to eat out of fear from the motivation to eat because we are hungry will bring you a long way toward coming into a complete balance of health and wellness. Become mindful of the stomach and lo and behold, you will reap humongous rewards.

One Bite at a Time

How much pleasure do you derive from eating delicious foods, or at least foods that are yummy to you? Speaking for myself, I derive endless pleasure from eating. My next question is how much time do you spend eating the delicious foods that you love to eat? How much time are you able to derive pleasure from eating?

Thanksgiving is a good example of what happens when we eat. Much time is spent in the kitchen by many people preparing the Thanksgiving meal. Hours are spent puttering and cooking and heating and shopping and preparing various dishes. Everyone sits down, typically a nice prayer or salutation is given for the entire family and then everybody gets down to the serious business of eating. Food is gobbled, one bite after another. Sometimes, talking completely stops for ten minutes. There is no necessity for one bite to be chewed and swallowed before the next is inserted into the mouth. And presto - after ten minutes each person around the table has successfully gobbled up as much as they can stomach.

Watch people carefully as they eat. Oftentimes you'll notice that a person will insert one bite into their mouth, chew once or twice and then insert a second bite, chew once or twice. They then insert a third, chew once or twice and finally, after four shovelfuls of food, they swallow. This is certainly not a mindful practice. What is also interesting is that we tend to eat the foods that we truly love – those foods with tastes that we treasure - more quickly than foods that do not offer as much pleasure.

The mindful practice and challenge this week is to slow down the process of eating. The challenge has a formula to it. I must warn you, it will take longer for you to eat each meal, but the benefits will be immeasurable. Here's the formula.

If you're eating with a utensil; a fork or a spoon, take the fork or the spoon and insert the food into your mouth. Then place the fork or the spoon down on the table and proceed to chew slowly, deliberately. Then and only then swallow.

After swallowing, pick up the utensil and do it one more time. No new food can be inserted until the existing food has been swallowed and its succulent treasures enjoyed. Fully and completely enjoy the tastes of each and every bite by proceeding with this small, short, simple formula—

1. *Insert the food into your mouth*
2. *Put the utensil down*
3. *Chew slowly and deliberately*
4. *Focus your attention on your mouth, not the plate or the spoon*
5. *Enjoy all the tastes and sensations*
6. *Swallow*
7. *Pick up the fork or the utensil from the table*

8. ***Proceed back to Step One***

If you are not eating with a fork or a spoon and if you are using your hands – for example if you're eating a sandwich or chips – the same applies. Take your item, whatever it might be, place it up to your mouth, take a bite and then put that sandwich or whatever you're holding in your hand down on your plate. Chew, swallow and then do it again one-bite-at-a-time.

This week, change your customary and habitual approach to eating. Focus your attention on your mouth. Enjoy the deliciousness of food that you love to eat.

Deeper Meaning Behind One Bite at a Time

The underlying meaning of the challenge to eat your food one bite at a time is actually profound. It introduces an awareness of the extent to which impatience or patience is a large part of your life. Do you have issues with impatience in your life?

If you have to wait in a long line to check out in a store, do you find yourself being particularly restless, unable to be present in the moment? If you are preparing a meal to eat, do you find yourself racing to the point of saying:

> *"I can't wait for this to be over because I have more things to do by the end of the day. The longer that I spend preparing this meal, the less time that I'll have to be able to do what it is that I want to actually accomplish today?"*

Are you then, a person who is persistently and continually impatient?

If this happens to be the case, it is probably more than likely also the case that you found the challenge to eat your food one bite at a time to be a horrendous challenge. Did you find that you got particularly impatient with being able to do this particular task? Most people do find it to be particularly challenging and difficult. Most people find that they are able to put their utensil down two or three

31

times but then, they sink back down into the same habitual way of eating and then by the end of the meal say,

> *"Oh, I forgot. That's right. I was supposed to put my utensil down between each and every full bite and swallow."*

It is in fact a difficult challenge, one that you will find will tickle your funny bone as you realize how difficult it is to honor and respect the challenge of being able to place your utensil down between each and every bite.

Let's go deeper. How impatient are you with your recovery process? Do you find yourself saying:

> *"I don't think I'm feeling any better this week than last. When am I going to be waking up and say whoa, I don't think I feel any symptoms at all; in fact I feel great?"*

Instead, you find that you wake up and there are certain symptoms that tend still to be present. Do you say to yourself,

> *"When is this going to lift? When is this going to lift – when is this going to lift?"*

In other words, are you impatient with your recovery process?

32

Guess what? If you are impatient, that is going to trigger the production of hormones that are not conducive to bringing your body back into full balance. You see, the impatience itself creates a problem with the recovery process.

The challenge of one bite at a time is a challenge of inviting you to slow it down, to become patient with each and every moment, to treasure the deliciousness of the experience, the tastes, the feeling, the texture of what it means to eat. It is a wonderful experience to ingest food into our bodies. Embellish that experience by making eating a mindful experience. This will transfer over into being more patient with each and every moment however it might unfold.

Becoming more patient expedites the process of recovery from any and all symptoms that you might currently be experiencing that happen to be associated with a diagnosis of Parkinson's disease.

Pay Attention to Your Tongue

Each week's challenge is crafted to direct your attention to places that are unfamiliar. This helps enforce mindfulness such that we are more mindful of our body's needs and what messages our body sends to us.

This week's challenge is to pay attention to your tongue. Really! That is your invitation this week. I bet you have never had an invitation like this one!

- *What is your tongue doing when you are eating?*
- *Does your tongue tend to hang out on the left side of your mouth or the right side of your mouth?*
- *Where does your tongue hang out when you swallow water?*
- *Does your tongue feel thick, mucousy, thin, slippery, tough, raggedy or edgy?*
- *How does your tongue feel from moment to moment during each and every day?*
- *Where does your tongue hang out in the moment when you are simply sitting, listening to someone else talk?*

Pay attention to your tongue this week especially when you eat. What is your tongue doing? How does your tongue feel? What is your tongue saying to you? Your tongue is typically a neglected body organ but it is also terribly essential to your health and well-being.

I'm quite sure this is not something you have done recently, so this exercise is guaranteed to place your attention on the present moment rather than focusing on the past or anticipating the future.

May you lead a stress-free life this week as you pay attention to what your tongue is doing in the moment.

Deeper Meaning Behind Paying Attention to Your Tongue

Admit it. Isn't the challenge of paying attention to your tongue as you eat a totally weird and wild invitation? After all, how many members of your family and how many of your friends have been focusing their attention on their tongue this week? Unless you involved others in this activity, my guess is you are the only one who happens to be paying attention to your tongue anywhere near or dear to you.

When we eat, it is common to dip into a repetitive space of thoughts, behaviors and actions that do not serve our best and highest good. The purpose of the mindfulness exercises is to make every effort to twist our way out of that endless trap of repetition that does not serve our best and highest good and to whisk away the negative thought forms that contribute to ill-health as we shift seamlessly into a positive space. After all, how benign can it be to simply pay attention to your tongue? Many of you may have discovered that it is actually a formidable challenge.

Think about another challenge that I certainly will never suggest. You can fantasize what it might require anyway. The task would be to construct a book of instructions to your tongue so your tongue would know precisely what it needed to do at any particular given moment. Now that book, even if it could be written, would be hundreds of thousands of pages long because the tongue is quite a

36

clever part of what our body does for us day in and day out.

Have you noticed that when you pay attention to your tongue, sometimes you begin to think -

> *"Well, I notice my tongue is slipped over to the right side, I wonder what's going to happen if I slip it over to the left side?*
>
> *I wonder how my tongue is related to my swallowing?"*

You see, without a tongue swallowing becomes incredibly difficult indeed.

The point of this task and all of the Parkinsons Recovery Series mindfulness exercises is to become totally present in the moment, to become aware of your body, to know precisely what your body is doing moment to moment and to become sensitive to what you are feeling. This, as it turns out, is the key to reducing stress. If we find ourselves in a typical mode of pondering over past mistakes or anticipating a tomorrow that may be worse than today, stress will accelerate. Acceleration of symptoms is inevitable.

There is a lesson to paying attention to the tongue that is actually quite profound. The hundreds of thousands of pages of a book that would be required to give instruction to the tongue would never be adequate. There would always be criticisms from one critic or another that the instructions were deficient. Your *Tongue Instruction* manual could never cover all the bases. The final and most magnificent lesson we can learn from paying close attention to our tongues is to:

"Celebrate the wonders and the miracle of the body."

Yes, the body really does know how to function. No, we really do not know how to give it instructions so that it functions any better than it knows how to do its job naturally and effortlessly. Our body is a miracle. Our body does know how to heal itself.

As you continue to pay attention to what your tongue is doing when you eat, listen, sit and talk, I invite you to also celebrate and honor the miracle of your body. It is indeed a divine creation composed of billions of cells that are healthy, vibrant, and doing precisely what they need to be doing for you moment to moment, day in and day out. As you focus your attention on your tongue, you will become more mindful of the present moment.

- **Notice how your stress dissolves.**
- **Celebrate the symptoms that dissolve.**
- **Honor the miracle of your body.**

History of the Food We Eat

Thanksgiving holiday is a celebration known particularly to individuals who live in America. Families gather together on a Thursday in November each year to gorge themselves with plates stacked high with food: cooked veggies, fruits, desserts. Oftentimes turkeys are involved because there is some connection to the history of the Pilgrims who first came to America.

The opportunity this week is put food on the center stage of your mindfulness practice. Elevate the role and importance of food just as happens during Thanksgiving holiday. This week, however, I invite you to give thanks to each bite of food that you ingest in a new and quite different way than is the custom Thanksgiving.

For each bite of food that you insert into your mouth, look back over the history of where that food originated. How did each and every bite of food get on your plate - ready to be retrieved and inserted into that precious, sacred vessel of your body?

What do I mean when I say look back into its history? Use the power of your imagination to acknowledge and honor all of the individuals that it took to serve food on your plate each meal this week.

For example, think of the:

- *Individuals who planted the seeds that started the growth process;*
- *Truckers who transported the food;*
- *Migrant workers - if they were involved - who harvested the food;*
- *Farmers and ranchers responsible for farming the food;*
- *Personnel at the packing plant;*
- *Grocers;*
- *Check out people at the grocers (if you purchased your food at the grocery store and had the food scanned by a human rather than a machine);*
- *Family members or other cooks who actually prepared the food.*

When you begin to search deeply into the history of the food that lands on your table each meal, it becomes quite amazing to realize the hundreds (if not thousands) of individuals who were required and needed to make meals happen for you.

Look back even farther. Acknowledge and honor the contribution of not just human beings but the bacteria, the fungi and even the bees that were needed to help the food grow into the form you now see on your plate. Treat the entire week as if each day were Thanksgiving. Before you

40

actually put the food into your mouth pause use the power of your imagination to:

- **Celebrate**
- **Honor**
- **Give thanks**

To each and every individual who made it possible for you to celebrate the delicious morsels you ingest during all meals of the week (whether you are eating on the run or casually at the dinner table).

Celebrate each day as if it were Thanksgiving Day as you give thanks not just to those persons in your immediate family (including yourself!) who had a role in bringing the food to the table but also to those

1. **Unseen**
2. **Unheard**
3. **Unknown**

Individuals and creatures that made it possible for you to have this very special opportunity to nourish your body mindfully.

Deeper Meaning Behind the Food We Eat

There is no doubt about it. The life force that is connected and associated with different foods varies greatly. Some foods contain little, if any, life force. They are colorless and lifeless. Because the food is essentially dead, we feel sluggish, fatigued and endlessly tired when we put that dead food into our body. Reflect back on how you feel when you eat fast food. My case rests!

Other foods are vibrantly colorful. They are replete with a life force that is boundless. In my hometown of Olympia, Washington, we have a Farmer's Market where there is a requirement that all of the food vendors make their food organically. When I pass by each of those stands, the colors in the food have an indescribable vibrancy. The food shouts out to those who pass by with joy and pride:

- *Look how pretty my colors are!*
- *Feel my strength!*
- *I can help you become well!*

If I happen to be a bit depressed or fatigued when walking through our local Farmer's Market, I can assure you that when I leave I am full of energy and enthusiasm. Even being close to food that has a vibrant life force is energizing and revitalizing.

Here is the way the energetic charge actually works. Every individual, every being who contributes to the creation and development and production of any food contributes to its "life force." When food is created with love, attention and mindfulness, we consume that full, delicious, energetic charge when we eat it. We feel vibrant inside.

For example, one of the reasons Thanksgiving is such a special holiday for so many individuals is that it turns out the Thanksgiving meal is made with love. It is made mindfully. It is a precious experience for all who are involved in bringing food to the table. In many households preparation of the actual meal may take five, six, even eight hours. The meal may only take 30 minutes to 45 minutes to actually consume. The feeling that everyone gets from eating that food may in part be,

> "I ate too much."

The feeling is also one of comfort, one of being inundated with a dose of love that is deliciously all-consuming.

Of course when food has a dark history, when perhaps it has been:

- *Genetically modified or*
- *Altered in some unnatural way*
- *Harvested in a cruel way*

43

The energetic charge is seriously depleted by the time it lands on our dinner plate to be eaten. .

Recognizing and acknowledging the history of where food comes from also acknowledges that we are all one. We are all connected to one another. We are all dependent on one another.

Of course, if you live in America, you probably have a sense of personal identity. We think of ourselves as independent beings rather than members of a group. This does not discount the reality that we are all connected.

In summary, the life energy of all who made the food possible that we enjoy (whether on Thanksgiving day or some other day) flows through us when we eat it. May you delight throughout the rest of the week in celebrating the majesty and the magic of what it means to consume food that is vibrant with energy and that energizes our life force. It is indeed a pleasure to be alive.

Has your work on these exercises been stress free? Has it been helpful in reducing your symptoms? I certainly hope so! This is the primary reason I developed the mindfulness exercises in the first place.

If you struggled with pacing out these mindfulness exercises so as not to induce more stress, there are several Parkinsons Recovery programs that might help expedite your recovery. My Parkinsons Recovery Mindfulness Program sends the mindfulness exercises in an email to you each and every week. The initial exercise is sent to your email address on day one of the week and the deeper implications are sent four days later. The Parkinsons Recovery Mindfulness Program takes one full year to complete as each exercise is introduced one week at a time. For more information visit:

www.stress.parkinsonsrecovery.com

Parkinsons Recovery Memberships involve a variety of support websites that are essential to recovery. A difference mindfulness exercise is posted each week. For more information on Parkinsons Recovery memberships visit:

www.parkinsonsrecovery.org

Of course, the approach that works for many people is to purchase a single volume of the Parkinsons Recovery

Mindfulness program at a time as you have already done! See the introduction for a listing of all nine Parkinsons Recovery Mindfulness volumes.

Thank you for Your Support

On behalf of the thousands of followers of Parkinsons Recovery, I want to thank you for your purchase of this booklet. One hundred percent (100%) of the profits purchases of my books and programs help subsidize the many free services I offer through Parkinsons Recovery -

www.parkinsonsrecovery.com

For information about other products, services and programs visit -

www.parkinsonsrecovery.me

www.ingramcontent.com/pod-product-compliance
Lightning Source LLC
Chambersburg PA
CBHW070232290526
45789CB00004B/1594